Weight Pain and Practical Wisdom for Weight Maintenance

Weight Pain and Practical Wisdom for Weight Maintenance

Helen P. Weeks

Library of Congress Control Number: 2009906051
ISBN: Hardcover   978-1-4415-4720-0
                 Softcover   978-1-4415-4719-4

This book was printed in the United States of America.

To order additional copies of this book, contact:
Xlibris Corporation
1-888-795-4274
www.Xlibris.com
Orders@Xlibris.com
50269

Contents

Dedication Page

This book is dedicated to my father (Churchill) Irwin Forte Wilkinson (Oct 16, 1927-May 4, 2002) whom, I knew, in his own way truly loved me.

Introduction

This semi-autobiographical book in 2 parts is unlike any other work you probably have read or will read. Book One—Weight Pain—is an accounting and unveiling of the events, traumas, fears, abandonment, rejections, ill-treatment, racism, rape, attempted rape and depression which has impacted the course of my life during my existence thus far. I just supply the examples. I change the names to protect the real people involved for their privacy. Beginning with my childhood, adolescence, teens and adulthood and in each case expanded my waistline in an attempt to comfort me, protect me, guard me and erect a bastion of defense from the outside forces and people that would otherwise confuse, torment and undermine my very existence and worth as a human being.

I evolved as an individual, guarded, scared and feeling alone and scattered by the same people I trusted and let in who, I thought, would love me, care for me, come to my aid and be there. So many times I was deceived, I was victimized, I was shamed into thinking that I did not count. I didn't matter. I was insignificant as a person, not worthy enough to be an individual or accepted for who I looked like or who I was. Or I was the nobody that nobody wanted. I decided to weed out the undesirables who came into my life. I decided to abandon the naysayers. I decided to be me, and to tailor my life to who and what I wanted to become. The weight pain was a lesson in the love of me to me, by me, for me. I decided what mattered; this would be my choice and mine alone. Society be damned. The weight pain of my life brought out the best in me. During the agony of the traumas, something was happening inside. I was becoming more determined to be assertive. I liked what I saw in me. I realized that the events which spanned my lifetime enriched me and enhanced me. I am what I am today because of my issues.

I thank God that I had the foresight and knowledge to look inside myself to unveil the hidden hurts. The weight pain that I suffered all those years freed me to become my best self. A self I love, respect and enjoy. I am fulfilled. I am happy. My life is wondrous. I say to you out there who are battling the bulge, try to free yourself as I have. Become who you really want to be. Change the imagery! Change the landscape! Change your essence! Identify the weight pain in your lives and let it go. You'll be glad you did.

Book two discusses ways in which you can take control over you. Simple daily things I suggest that can help take the edge off. I give an account of how you can re-evaluate the world around you in order to facilitate and ease your day to help accommodate, sustain and manage your weight. Many of these ideas you have probably heard of or thought about but have not seriously considered implementing them. Well, maybe now is the time. Use the ideas contained herein to help you achieve your goals and whatever you establish for yourself. I did and have learned through my life experience what really matters to me.

If some of the text contained herein may seem disconnected, disjointed, fragmented or even illogically sequenced, it is merely the way that I remember it.

Book I

Weight Pain

I have been alone all my life. I learned very early in childhood that I had to take care of me. I learned probably at 2 ½ years of age at the time of my rape that I was going to be it. I can still see the room. I can still smell the bed. I know what I was wearing. I still feel the banging against me. The house, the yard, the surroundings are very vivid in my mind's eye. I will never forget this. This was the first day that trust would elude me for a goodly portion of my life. It was in those moments that, even as a 2 ½ year old, I knew something was terribly wrong. Terribly!

My mother had gotten a job and a friend of the family, Miss Carol would be the babysitter. She had two sons. I don't remember their names, just what they smelled like. I remember the rooms being dark and shaded. Drab with no brightness. I remember the backyard with a tent that also smelled like stale, damp blankets. The food she gave us was crap. For breakfast, we'd be served cold rice with milk which was horrible. My sister Evie who was two years older told my mother what it was like there and she never worked again. My father turned Earline into a homemaker.

The images from those days are stamped in my brain. I guess it's true that you don't forget the traumas in your life. And this is where the weight pain begins.

I wasn't born fat. I was a cute, chubby, chocolate brown baby girl who weighed five pounds and eight ounces at birth. I started out with, what would have been considered at that time in 1948 as normal or average. I had big, brown eyes and lots of curly hair. I was adorable, but that was destined to change.

Events in my early childhood would take over and consume my life. I also felt that I had no protection. I had no support, not even from my parents. As I child, I suffered from nightmares. I always wanted to sleep with someone to spare myself the horrors of the night. I hated sleeping alone. I remember once, about age five, going into my parents' room for some comfort and I was chased away. I guess that was the real beginning of the end. I saw them cuddled up and desperately wanted part of that, but it was not to be had. I went back to my bed and lay awake all night, too afraid to close my eyes. I was a victim of night terrors, which lasted years and years. One night, I even begged my mother's brother, my Uncle Frankie to sleep with me. He finally relented. I got a good night's sleep. I felt totally detached from my parents and from that moment on, I never again felt close to them. In my mind, I had been abandoned and I did not know why. Irwin and Earline were not having any late night visitors under any circumstances.

I was in the world looking out, never feeling that I was in it, together with the rest of the people in my life. My sister Evie and I were close as kids, but I couldn't sleep with her, either. We had twin beds and there wouldn't really be enough room. Besides, she was the neat one and I was the slob. Oscar and Felix shared a bedroom with a string down the middle at times. We had a fight once, and I picked up a knife. I don't think Evie really knew I was tormented with nightmares. At times, she was a little indifferent. We loved each other, but as we grew up, we started to move apart. I couldn't figure out for the life of me why no one was on my side. Was I the bad child? Was I the bad person?

I remember once when my mother had a party, some of her friends were in our bedroom sitting around and I kept calling her because I needed her and someone said "Go away!" I will never forget that.

I look back on my childhood to see where the feelings of love were and I can't find them. I know in my head that my mother and father loved me. But I didn't feel it. They never said it. My parents were not demonstrative. I craved affection.

My father worked in New York City as a building superintendent on East 11th Street and University. He got that job soon after his discharge from the Army. He actually started working in a store called United Farms on the corner of University and East 11th, then graduated into being building superintendent. At first, he had a few houses, then over time, that number grew to include houses on East 10th Street as well. My father was so well liked and adored by the homeowners that he was dubbed "The Mayor of East 11th Street." I would occasionally go to his job between the ages of seven and nine.

One Sunday, my mother dressed me up and I went to my father's main building at 16 East 11th Street. There was a French restaurant across the street and they were making some sort of film. There was a beautiful blonde woman with the most gorgeous blue eyes sitting in the back of a carriage (they gave carriage rides). Because my father knew the owners, I got to sit next to the lady and the film director said to me "Don't look at the camera." I felt so pretty and beautiful, just like she must have. That was one of the most special times in my life. Until a lady named Nellie told me that my father was also the father of her two children, a boy and a girl.

For a little girl my age, I was hit with a ton of bricks. I was already battling with the man who was my father. I was already trying to find ways for him to love me, and now this. What was I supposed to do? I don't know. I had two other siblings. Where were these people? Where did they live? What were their names? I later met the boy, Bernie. He was a baby toddler. I remember going over to this lady's house and she was doing her laundry. I offered to help hang up the clothes and I never did it before. After I finished, when she looked out the window, she laughed. She thought the way I hung the clothes was the funniest thing. The distance between my father and myself grew. I think, subconsciously, I started to hate him. I began to realize that as I grew older, that my father had two homes and two families. My father would be gone for two or three days a week, every week. One of my friends said to me once (we lived in the Marcy Houses), when she saw me run to my father, "Helen, that's your father; we didn't know you had a father." That's because he was a part time dad. He was spending his time on the job or with other people.

I had another episode at about age seven with one of my mother's friends. As I said, we lived in the Marcy Houses in the Williamsburg section of Brooklyn. It was on the edge of the Hasidic Jewish community. The Marcy Houses were built at the end of the Second World War to help house the returning soldiers and to promote low income housing resulting from the Depression. My parents moved in when I was two months old. The idea was to integrate the housing complex with two white and two black families on every floor. That would be the case until the whites started moving out to suburbia. It would be a world and life experience unmatched by any other.

The Marcy Houses turned out to be a prison within a prison, The idea was to house thousands of families in what was called "the projects," but it became a life sentence of debauchery, crime loss of ethics, values, morality and ultimately a dirty, infested, pitiless vortex spinning out of control where hopelessness, despair and addiction would reign forever. The physical environs would become as barren and bleak as outer space.

Family life would dissipate over time and the nuclear family would stand in time as a once-taken snapshot. Unwed mothers would paint the landscape with strollers, absentee fathers would become unemployed, jailed or the local drug dealers. The whites, by now would be long gonetheir flight would have soared into the cleaner, safer suburbs. I witnessed this demise and decay before we left, just before its peak. In the late 1960s, the host of families I saw destroyed became strained by alcoholism, rampant crime, marital infidelity and destruction. My waistline was in disarray as was my community.

At the time, my mother had a full swing party life with some of the locals: Miss Flossie, Miss Evelyn, Miss Ruthie, Miss Lisa, Miss Richardeen, Mr. Ernest and the one man who made me take down my panties and expose myself to him. Where was my mother? She went to the store and left him there to watch me while she was gone. He didn't touch me physically, but his eyes molested me as he leered over my so-called "private parts" in the nude.

And the lessons of mistrust abound. I was getting the message loud and clear that these people were not to be trusted. So far, it was Miss Carol's son, my father, this sicko and now Dinky. On the top floor of my grandparents' building was a family of two boys. I was now about ten or eleven. One day, Dinky's mother went to do the laundry while we were in the apartment. All of a sudden, Dinky started grabbing me into the small side room, next to what we called the piano room, in my grandma's house. He was laughing all the while pulling at my clothes as he got on top of me to rape me. I was dumbfounded. When I realized what was about to happen, his mother came back. I was saved. That ended my friendship with Dinky, who was, by the way, sixteen or seventeen. I was a child playing with someone I thought I could trust.

I was growing chubby. I was size 12 ½ as a young girl. I was eating everything in sight. At 12 years of age, I weighed 126 pounds; by 16, I was 160. The weight pain was in full swing. The rape, the attempted rape, my father's second family were all adding up. The rejection, confusion and mistrust were all hitting their stride.

I had learned thus far that you could not trust people in your inner circle, family, friends or otherwise. That you must learn to be guarded, at all cost. That you cannot let people in anymore, because they will hurt you. You had to take charge to protect yourself. The weight was just a way to do that. I had to lose my desirability. I had to retreat inward. I had to become invisible.

Even though in my head I could not trust these people, I still searched for love and validation. Chops, or Donald Kemp would be my first love. At sixteen, I lost my virginity. Donald was a "man about town." He bedded quite a few girls in the neighborhood. Mazy Pinckney was one of them while we were together. I knew, but I didn't want to know. I needed someone for me. And at this time in my life when my father was absent most of the time, Donald was what the doctor ordered. We had sex every chance we got. I called his house every day hoping that his mother, Miss Joanne, had a housecleaning job or something. I wanted to be with him more than anything in this world. Until it was time to graduate high school and Donald had no ambition to aspire to greatness, so, I ended the relationship.

The "War of the Worlds" between my parents never stopped. My mother cried at least four or five times a week due to my father's mistreatment. Her main complaint was his lack of attention and care for her. His being away a lot bothered her tremendously. I was left with carrying the weight. I was left with the role of "filling in" because of his absence. I had to do everything for my mother. I had to take her shopping; I had to do all the small repairs; I had to be her left hand as well as her right. I had to be her friend, confidant, listener, counselor and, ultimately, her caregiver. I loved my mother and would absolutely do anything for her. She had to know that in this life, she would always have her daughter Helen, even if no one else was ever there. And so it was. I never abandoned my mother as others in her life had. And the weight pain continued.

Earlene got lucky one night and became pregnant with my brother who was born in 1964. My mother thought that after my brother Eric was born that things would change. They did not. It was our lives as usual. You ask, where was Evie in all this? She was around somewhere. I guess she didn't want to see or just couldn't see the reality. Her childhood memories veered elsewhere. Irwin was the invisible, the elusive, the un-dad.

Eric would also grow up with the pain as well as the knowledge that Irwin was not in the father mode. We can look back at Irwin's life as a child. But, we know very little about that since Irwin did not talk to us. He didn't talk to us about anything. You need to be home to do that. So, Eric, as well as myself, went unlovedor at least we felt unloved. Irwin was not the demonstrative typeor at least not the touchy-feely type. I cannot remember Irwin ever kissing me or telling me that he loved me. I am almost certain that Eric never experienced the same. Evie can speak for herself.

I do remember going to my father's job at 16 East 11ᵗʰ Street to see him. There was a dark-skinned young girl in the doorway with him. He must have told her something to get her to leave, since she hurried off. I didn't ask him who she was when I approached; I knew I wouldn't believe him. I knew he was living a lie, a big lie. After my encounter with that little person, I seldom went there. Besides, he didn't want any of us there anyway.

I did learn a few things about Irwin only after I asked him. I don't really know why I asked. I just did. He told me that he was called "Churchill" in his youth because he was good at playing pool. Also that while he was in the Army when in Germany near the end of the Second World War, as soon as the Germans saw the black soldiers coming at them, they dropped their guns and ran.

I adore my sister Evie. When we grew up, we were partners in crime. Mischief was our middle name. One morning, we sat under the kitchen table eating sugar from the sugar bowl and our mother caught us. Earline took no prisoners. We were, of course, punished. I guess we were about five and seven at the time. On another occasion, we collected cigarette butts, tore up strips of brown paper, rolled our own cigarettes with the left over tobacco, under the kitchen table, smoking our little selves away. "Eagle eye Earline" was on the case. This time we each got a spanking. Evie and Helen were as "thick as thieves." As children growing up in our pre-teen years, we were inseparable. Evie was named after our maternal grandmother, Evella, and I was named after our paternal grandmother, Helen. We loved these women with all our hearts, both of whom were as doting as grandmothers can be. We were spoiled rotten. Grandmother Helen made us aprons out of my grandpa's old shirts to cover our pretty dresses. She would also make us the best break fasts in the world. Farina or Wheatena® with sweet and condensed milk, sweet buttered toast or franks fried in butter on the big coal stove. She lived in a nine room railroad flat at 1031 Bedford Avenue in Brooklyn. That was one of the most fun places we ever spent during the summer. Grandma Helen also taught us our very first prayer. "Now I lay me down to sleep, I pray the Lord my soul to keep. If I should die before I wake, I pray the Lord my soul to take." I celebrate her birthday every year on October 2. I know in my heart, that she loved me dearly. I felt her love as a child. I even hum as she did. Grandma also read the Bible every day.

However, when she passed on, I felt abandoned. Grandma Helen had a stroke. She could have lived, but she did not want to; she just let go. I was heartbroken. I felt part of me died with her. She had been my rock. She had been one of the few people I knew who really loved me and now she was gone. I was so unhappy. One night, I cried for her and she came to me and said that everything would be all right. I felt better. I had been teaching a few years now and was trying to fit in.

Evella Jackson was a superstar. She had a restaurant. She was a nurse. She owned real estate. She was a seamstress, milliner, clothing designer and one of the kindest people in my life. Grandma Becky as she was also known made our Easter outfits, coats, dresses and, at times, our hats in a place where she lived called "the shop," on Tompkins Avenue in Brooklyn. It was thought there was nothing this lady could not do. My sister and I idolized her as though she was royalty.

Grandma Evella wrote me her last letter before she passed. She had become unhappy with her life and was reaching out to me, her "chug-a-lug." That was a name she gave me as a child, since I was so chubby. She, too, loved me so much.

Aunt Jean, Aunt La La (Lois), both Grandmas, Aunt Millie were all gone. Evie and I would soon move in different directions. We went to different high schools, had different friends and we would eventually lead vastly different lives.

Evie married Norman Douglas Crooke, "Butchie." She was madly in love with him. Butchie had been in the Army and was settling into life back in the Marcy Houses. After awhile, he and Evie married. They had the cutest little girl named Dana Sharisse, who was a preemie, born January 15, 1968. She had to stay in the hospital for a bit until she gained enough weight to come home. Evie and Butchie were so happy. Married life kept Evie busy with her new family especially after she moved out to Coney Island. She eventually gave birth to Norman DeShawn Crooke, born November 24, 1976. As for me, I had to endure more weight pain.

Charles Foy was my mother's friend. He was married to a witch, or at least, that was what I thought. They lived in the projects somewhere and had two boys. One was Donny. I met him once. Charles was the closest thing I had to a real father. He did everything for us and my mother. He came over so much that one time I actually called him "Daddy." He gave me my first nickname, "Lump Lump." I was a chubby little girl and he adored me. When he and my mother stopped seeing each other, I was crushed. They broke up when my mother became pregnant with my brother. Charlie wanted my mother to leave my father, but she wouldn't. I wish she had. I would have had a real daddy. I felt Charlie's love for me.

I didn't know my real father loved me until after I became a teacher. I was over 25 years of age when I found this out. I went to his job again and one of the tenants was leaving the building just as I entered and my father introduced us. This lady knew everything about me: where I taught, grade levels, everything! I stood there speechless. In that moment, after all those lonely years, I finally realized that Irwin loved Helen. He had to, why else would he spend so much time talking about me? But it was too little, too late. The damage was already done.

My childhood, although filled with lots of activities, missed one essential ingredient which would have made me whole. My father never praised me, never hugged me, never touched me and barely supported us (My mother got lots of money from Charles Foy.).

I started working my junior year of high school and I have supported myself ever since. My first job was at Key Food, a local supermarket. Then it was off to F. W. Woolworth's until I went to college.

The scarcity of my father weighed heavily on me every day of my life.

Aunt Jean was the nuttiest relative we had in the family. She was rambunctious, raucous and a raving lunatic. But we loved her. She was a doting aunt. She had no children of her own even though she was married to "Uncle Buster." Her alias was "Honey Tubbs," and boy was Honey a mess. One evening, Aunt Jean was found walking home from Tom's Bar, the local watering hole in a black bathing suit with no shoes on her feet. My friends were hysterical with laughter and teased me no end. Aunt Jean was the talk of the town. I remember her saying once, in regards to men, "I can't stand 'em." You see, Aunt Jean, too, was a rape victim. Her father, my maternal grandfather, William "Happy" Jackson had done the dirty deed and had been locked away in an insane asylum. This was the family's secret. No one ever talked about this until after Aunt Jean died. Then my mother told me everything. She always did. In retrospect, I can see the pain in her. I could sense her anger. She was a drinker and a Hell raiser and now I know why. Aunt Jean died of complications of heart failure. She grieved over this since she was 16 years old, the time the dirty deed had taken place. She never recovered from it. How she happened to marry Leland (Buster) Tubbs remains a mystery.

(There was another rape in the family, but I cannot go into it. I need to protect the person.)

The childhood years were quite traumatic at times. I wore a mask, grew my waist line as a shield, a plate of armor, a barrier against the agony and angst which plagued me. I became shy and withdrawn and no one even noticed, no one. My world was such a scary and frightening place. There I was, alone, drifting and living in a state of total confusion.

Life was full of rejection. It was everywhere. People were cruel to one another, hurtful and, at times, just plain rude. I used to think that I was born in the wrong century and somehow there was a mistake. I was transfixed in an era or age that I just didn't belong in.

Blackness and being black was a curse. It was a denial of one's humanity, as denial of one's existence. It was being in an abyss of a no man's land. Everywhere I seemed to turn, I was being bombarded with being black and being undesirable, unwanted and unappreciated.

I went to John Ericsson Junior High School in Greenpoint, Brooklyn. It was on Meserole Avenue. The neighborhood was filled with white Slavic people. We had to walk from the train station about four or five flocks to the school. That was the worst walk we had to take. The white kids called us nigger, blackie and looked at us with such disdain and hatred, which made me sick to my stomach. Yes, those early sixties were a real killer. Literally! My spirit was being chipped away every day of my life as I attended that school. The teachers were brutal, too. Mrs. Styles, my math teacher was as racist as she could be. I never did well in math because she ignored me everyday. She would never acknowledge my presence or abilities. I did the best I could and passed. Mr. Battaglia, my typing teacher, sat all the black kids in the back and never paid any attention to us either. And, to this day, I am a poor typist. However, the one saving grace was Albert Weiner, my social studies teacher. He called me "Marble Mouth" because I spoke so rapidly, you could hardly understand what I was saying. But he was a great teacher and he inspired me to go further in life. On open school night, he told my mother that I could be anything I wanted because I was a bright girl. And I will never forget Albert Weiner.

John Ericsson had its redeeming qualities, though. There was my English teacher, Mrs. Sunshine. That's right, her name was "Sunshine," and shine she did. Mrs. Sunshine was a stout woman with wavy black hair and when she smiled, she lighted up the room. She was just adorable. She spoke with such clarity and authority that you dared not cross her in any way. You just did what she told you to do. In other words, she took no prisoners and everyone knew it.

I hated gym. By now, I was a real "Chubbette" and weighed in at 140 pounds on my 5 foot, 3 inch frame. My gym teacher, a black woman, would chuckle to herself because I could not do the rollovers and other exercises she demanded of us. I remember wanting to just get up and walk out, but that was a no-no! So, I prevailed! I received a C in gym.

I went to Washington Irving High School in New York City. Luckily for me, it was an all-girls school. No boys, no trauma. It was a piece of cake.

College, on the other hand, was a real eye opener. Racism was like a disease that everyone on campus seemed to have. Queens College back in 1967, in the midst of the Civil Rights Movement was a real challenge. Some of my professors were real jerks. One I can recall embarrassed me in front of the entire class when he asked me, "How did a black girl like you get Wilkinson as a last name, it's English?" I didn't answer, of course, I just looked at him like the idiot he was.

There was a lot of heat and tension on campus during that time and some of the more outspoken white students would take it upon themselves to verbally assault the black students. I had such an event. This unassuming white boy approached me and said, "The only things you black people will ever get is what we give you." "We" meaning, of course, white folks. I said, "Well, we'll see, won't we?" And I walked away.

I was getting clobbered on all fronts with this "black thing." But I never expected it within my own community, the black community. My paternal family hailed from the Caribbean, specifically Trinidad and Barbados, with some intermarriage with Jamaicans. My paternal grandmother's side of the family were light skinned with nice hair. I had cousins, her sister's daughter's children, Lynn and Brenda. They were two of the most stuck up, color struck people of my childhood. We had an affair at my Uncle Otto's house—we were celebrating the birth of his first child, my cousin Laura. The two of those cousins, looked at my sister and myself, their little darky cousins, and ignored us the entire evening. They didn't come near us. They treated my sister and I as though we were lepers. And, of course, no one noticed. But I did. I was twelve years old.

Denise Elston was a beautiful very, very fair black girl with fire red hair and freckles. She grew up in the projects with her family suggesting humble beginnings like the rest of the people from the projects. We ended up going to Queens College together years later. At Queens College, there was this very handsome, but very dark-skinned boy, Curtis, who was head-over-heels in love with Denise. He wanted desperately to take her to a campus party. He asked us, a few of her friends, to tell her on his behalf because he was so shy, so we did. Her immediate response was, "Oh, he's too dark, he'll clash with my skin." I was floored! Needless to say, they didn't go.

Peggy was also a light, bright campus darling. She was "high yellow," with long stringy "good hair," and ugly. It didn't matter. The guys were all over her. I could not compete. I never had a boyfriend or dated anyone from Queens College.

My best friend Karen and I took a trip to Washington, DC to see the musical Shenandoah at the Kennedy Center for the Performing Arts one weekend. We got all gussied up, looking as fine and cure as we could be. We went to this club, which shall remain nameless, to party hearty. We sat and we sat and we sat. Finally, this handsome dark skinned brother came over to us and introduced himself. He then said "Ladies, look around, what do you see?" We then realized that everyone in the place was light, bright and cream-colored. What a revelation. No one was asking the "darkies" to dance no matter how "fine" we thought we looked. Walter suggested we follow him to another club. So we went. It was a huge warehouse down by the water. You could hear the music two blocks away as you approached,

thumping and bumping. When we entered, looked around, everyone
was crispy, burnt, chocolate or charcoal having a blast. We partied
until dawn.

That same weekend, Murphy's Law would prevail, as I ran into
an old friend, Hugh Mattson. Spoke to him; he denied me. He told
me that I was mistaken. He said everyone confuses him with this
person. I knew High from the Marcy Projects. He had a brother
Richard who was a friend of my sister's who frequented our home.
Hugh just didn't want to be seen in public talking to a "little darky"
from his distant past.

The early seventies were tumultuous. It seemed that no matter
where I turned, the sky was falling. I was in the early years of my
teaching career at Huntington High School on Long Island, New
York. I had come to the school when a young teacher named Morris
Brandon had just up and quit one Friday afternoon. I was just
terminated at Walt Whitman High School because a teacher on
sabbatical had decided to return mid-year. I was hired to teach at
Huntington High School that same day.

The climate at Huntington was a little chilly. The racial tension had
not yet melted down. The area in South Huntington had been looking
for black teachers to help ease and quell some disruptions that had
taken place, so I was told. The staff, at first, wasn't too friendly. Only
a few extended a hand of fellowship. I remember walking down the
hall and feeling invisible as no one would speak to me. It was even
worse in the faculty lounge and cafeteria. Up close, I had no idea that
white folks could be so cruel and alarming to one another. I was so
scared and off balance most of the time. In my classroom, the white
kids challenged me to no end. They wanted to make sure that I wasn't
a "token nigger" who really had no expertise as a history teacher. So,
I had to up my game on all fronts. I gained thirty pounds.

Things started to balance out. Some people mellowed and
friendships grew, but my waistline remained intact. By now, the
district had hired a few more black teachers and had hired an
assistant principal who was coming in from the south. His name was
Bill Samuelson. The school nurse, Ellen Worth, thought that I should
meet him and she told me about him. Well, he must have seen me
first, and his comment to another black person was "she's too fat and
too dark for me." You see, Mr. Samuelson was a light, bright, tall, slim
man who had a penchant for the high yellow or white types and I just

didn't fit the bill. That was a blow. I guess I would have clashed with his skin and body type. What's a girl to do? I never let him know that I was told of his comment. I still gave him respect and spoke to him every time I saw him. Yet, I was still stabbed in my heart by his open and pronounced rejection.

Eventually, I decided to lose weight because I liked David Washington. David was a special education teacher, patient, kind and loved his job. David was tall, lean, handsome, intelligent and fun to be with. But there was one requirement to be with him. I had to lose weight. So I dropped eighty pounds and the romance was on. I fell head-over-heels in love with David, but he was not in love with me. I was blinded by the thought of David, the touch of David, the smell of David and the everything of David. Then it was over. He took me out to lunch one day and told me that he was getting married. The signs had been all around, but I just wouldn't let them in, I couldn't, as it would just be too painful, it would hurt too much. It did. I took a long time to fall out of love with David, but I learned one very important thing in the process. Never lose weight to get a man. It's only the body they want and not the person. You're left with a hole in your soul that you fill right back up.

During this period of thinness, my building principal took a shot at me also. Larry Babcock stood at the counter every morning in the main office as you walked in to greet you. When I came in, I got a special hello: his tongue. He would slyly roll his tongue at me while squinting his beady little eyes. This went on for days and days. Even at the school prom. I had a date; my friend Luther took me. It didn't matter. Larry made me so uncomfortable at the table that I had to get up and leave. Larry finally got the message. It was a no. A resounding NO!

Male teachers floated past my room daily. I was a fox. I was gorgeous. The attention was killing me. I couldn't take it. I wasn't used to it. I had to get rid of it. I gained all the weight back. The attention disappeared and I was relieved.

My life was bitter, sour, dark, drab. Little light shined through my days. I was hiding inside myself daily. I was alone, scared and felt hopeless, depressed and thought of suicide. The world turned out to be an unfamiliar place, awkward, desolate and impenetrable. People . . . men were everywhere, but they seemed to keep their distance. Or at least they didn't want any part of me, intimately, except as a sex object. Smiling faces were plastic, stunted and tempered with falsehoods. I was feeling hollow inside. I was going home to madness. My mother was a crier. She cried all the time. My father was the culprit. Absentee Irwin struck again and again. When he came home, he ignored my mother. He didn't sleep in the same room. He had the middle room which used to be my old room before I moved to the second floor. Irwin was quiet. He didn't say two words to anyone. He slept and slept. He watched TV and slept. In the meantime, my mother cooked his food and placed it on the table like the dutiful wife that she was. There was no relationship between Irwin and Earline. In the early years of their marriage they would fight. Until one day he hit her, she picked up an iron and swung it at him and he didn't hit her again for a long, long time. I was about five or six at that time. That fight took place in the bathroom. We lived in the Marcy Houses back then.

Things really did not change much between my parents. My mother told me that my grandmother made my mother and father get married. She already had my sister Evie, and when she got pregnant again with me my grandmother lowered the boom and made her get married. I guess that's when the trouble started. Irwin punished Earline from that day on. Even though there would be good times, it would be obvious, Irwin really didn't love Earline. He would be trapped in a loveless marriage.

My father was forty thousand dollars in debt at age 72. Where had that money gone? It was not in my mother's house. The money had gone to the other family. He had not spent it on her or on us. He bought my mother used furnishings all her life. I bought my mother her first brand new living room set after my marriage to Alan. My sister and I helped our parents refinance their home and pay off the debt.

As my parents aged, Irwin began to mellow out but my mother's health started to worsen. The pain and agony she suffered all those years finally took its toll. She had heart disease, high blood pressure, depression and dementia. My father never went to the doctor. He died May 4, 2002 of a stroke. He was 74.

It's funny, strange, how after someone dies you learn something critical about their past. Something you find worth knowing, something you could have been proud to know, something you could have acknowledged earlier, especially in one's youth. I had to go through my father's personal effects, which were in the basement. He had a small safe, a medium sized blue plastic box which contained Abraham Lincoln wheat backed pennies, a collection dating from 1909 to 1965. He also had a picture of his father, Otway L. Wilkinson in his Fraternal Mason Brotherhood regalia. The most enlightening find, though, were his honorable discharge papers from the United States Army.

This is to certify that
Irwin F. Wilkinson PA42 278 351 Private
Company D1321, Engineers Construction Group
Army of the United States
Is hereby honorably discharged from the military service of the
United States of America
This Certificate is awarded as a testament of honest and
Faithful service to this country.

Given at Separation Center
    Fort Dix, New Jersey

Date: 5 February 1947

It also contained from the Army of the United States: The separation qualification record gave an account of his military occupational specialty which was six months of rifleman, four of duty soldier, grade private. There was also a summary of his military occupation. Rifleman 745: used rifle, pistol and art of concealment during infantry training while stationed in Korea. Fired at dummy targets, also patrolled warehouses, depots and guarded at military installation entrances where personnel passes were checked.

As I read these documents, I wished he had shared this with me. I wished that I could have visualized him in action as a small child or seeing my daddy holding a rifle, shooting at the enemy. But it was not to be and I would pay the price.

At the Lawrence H. Woodward Funeral Home, his side of the family sat in the back and kept to themselves. We (that is, my sister and myself) had to go back there to visit with them while my mother sat up front. It was so hurt, but I put up a good front. I was grieving. My mother was grieving. We were full of pain. I was full of pain. My life had been full of turmoil and it was not over, even at this funeral. My father's family was clueless about what my mother had been through. They had no idea how she had suffered.

I went to live with my mother in Brooklyn, New York. I was going through a lot. I was miserable, but my mother needed me more than what I was experiencing. I could not fail her. We left. My finances were a shambles. I had lost my bookstore, my home, divorced my husband after being an abused wife, dealt with mega lawsuits, I had to rent a house, break the lease, my son was depressed and failing in school, my total world had collapsed. All this took place between 1991 and 1997. I gained another thirty pounds.

I had been hiding all my pain and agony from everyone until Ronald Baer. He was the Social Studies Department Chair. One night, he had a party and I went. He walked me to my car and I unloaded on him like a ton of bricks. I told him what I was going through in my marriage with my husband and how he was treating me and my daughter. I left him speechless. To this day, no one knows the real story of how he abused my children and I suffered at the hands of one Alan R. Weeks. I found a way to get rid of that monster and I took it. You wonder, why did I marry such a person? He was a liar, a very good liar. He perfected a persona that was impeccable, foolproof, believable before the marriage, but it began to unravel after the nuptials. In retrospect, I was gullible, stupid, hungry for someone to love me and I didn't stop to smell the roses. I just grabbed them and kept on going. It cost me more than I can say.

My life with Alan was one of terror and fear. He was at first a real charmer. He was sweet, brilliant, a genius and someone who could hold a conversation, read a book and watch TV all at the same time. The real reason is that I got pregnant with my son Christopher. I knew the exact moment of conception. I knew it was a boy. I knew I was keeping him. I knew I was in trouble.

Alan and I married on the fateful day of July 20, 1986. I call it fateful because it was meant to be. I have come to know this through my experience that there are no coincidences in this world. Things that happen are meant to be. My life with Alan was full of lessons to be learned for my growth and spiritual development. In retrospect, I owe him a lot and thank him for who he helped me become today. I can enumerate the gory details of our marriage and have you all in tears, but what purpose would that serve? Alan has come full circle.

He has grown in so many ways and has become a much better person. We were separated for fourteen years and our divorce became final in 1996. There are still many fences to be mended but we are working on those and my children still need to overcome many of the traumas from the marriage. Especially my daughter Heidi who suffered the most. Alan's treatment of her at times was abominable to say the least. But she bravely with her wits and smarts weathered the many stormy days and nights. The one good thing Alan did for her was to teach Heidi to read and she became a voracious reader at five years old, reading as many as twenty-five children's books a week. Heidi grew up to be a nuclear engineer in the U. S. Navy.

I moved to Mesa, Arizona in April 2004 and guess who was living here, too? Alan Weeks, my ex-husband. Now, how's that for fate? And, yes, we are best buddies. He has changed so much and is doing so much better. I am so proud of him. He is still a little nutty (he always was). My son Christopher has mixed feelings about all of this, but is willing to take things one day and one step at a time since he was the one who sought out Alan in the first place. Christopher found Alan on line and asked him where he lived and voila! We occasionally have family time together which is nice, but it is still hard for us to leave the horrors of the past behind. I, for one, still remember his hands around my neck trying to strangle me and the bottle of wine he smashed to smithereens on the kitchen counter one morning, or missing door knobs, phones, locked windows the night he planned to kill us. The yoyo dieting that took me up sixty pounds had made me a nervous wreck. Yet my children and I have prevailed. We have survived. Alan has made his amends and I forgave him.

After my tumultuous marriage was over, I really began to pour myself into my teaching. It was my second self, outside of my children and my home. I had always believed that there were two places in life that you had to have true happiness. One was at home, the other was at work. This belief was part and parcel to my sanity. My home life had been out of balance, out of kilter for such a while that my classroom was on the brink of destruction. I was struggling, balancing the two, but the fight I waged to do was so grounded in my determination to win that I did win and I continued to be the master teacher of my dreams. The powerhouse I was meant to be. I was a force to be reckoned with. My mind went on full throttle ahead. I lost sixty pounds and enjoyed the best teaching of my career. The burden had been lifted, or so I thought.

After I put Alan out in 1991, the walls caved in. There were the financial hardships to endure. I was being sued by my former landlord where I had my bookstore. The balloon payment on the building mortgage was past due; my home mortgage went into foreclosure since it was collateral for the building. I was in a lawsuit with George Caico who was tenant in my building at 718 New York Avenue in Huntington, New York. George and I had a bitter history which consisted of his not paying rent or paying for the building after he agreed to buy it from me. I was nearly $500,000 in debt. But I was fortunate to have two of the best lawyers on my cases, Jeffrey Waller and Anthony Conforti. Both of these men worked *pro bono* for me, which was a miracle. I will forever be indebted to these great human beings.

Alan had been hiding the mail from me while I was working. My landlord's attorney was sending me all kinds of paperwork that I was not receiving. I was also being sued by a Mr. Nottman to whom Alan had sold forgeries, the former owner of our bookstore, Polyanthos Green Street Books, hence the nightmare continued and the pounds added up.

On December 15, 1997, I had to file chapter 7 with the United States Bankruptcy Court, Eastern District of New York.

My life in Arizona turned out to be one of the best decisions I ever made. I came here after making a mother-daughter trek cross country with my daughter Heidi in December 2003. Heidi was in the Navy and had to drive her car to San Diego where she was stationed and had a ten day leave. It was an awesome drive. The country, which I had never seen west of the Mississippi, or New Jersey, for that matter, was absolutely beautiful. When we arrived in Arizona, it was breathtaking. I was disabled from my car accident in 2002 which left me with chronic low back pain, facet syndrome, nerve damage to my neck, shoulders and right arm. I could no longer tolerate cold and damp weather, nor could my mother. Back in New York, we were both shut-ins. Arizona, however, seemed like paradise, so a move was imminent. I told my doctor that I felt so much better in Arizona and he suggested that I move to a warmer climate. That February, my son and I engaged a realtor, flew to Arizona and moved into our new home on June 30, 2004. I thanked God every day for this blessing.

My son Christopher slowly adjusted to Arizona life. From Huntington, New York to Brooklyn, New York and now Mesa, Arizona in a little more than just two years was quite painful. He did not know which end was up. He was still fighting depression, confusion, loneliness and despair. He had attended three schools: Huntington High School, Bishop Loughlin High School, Harry Van Arsdale High School and now Desert Ridge High School. He would be repeating tenth grade. Christopher rose to the challenge. It took perseverance, tough love, stamina and lots of faith and prayers. He graduated high school with the biggest smile on his face. Mine, too.

My daughter Heidi is one of the loves of my life. She is brilliant. She is a little genius. She was so smart as a baby, she scared me. When I brought her home from the hospital, I had the most beautiful crib with all the trimmings ready and waiting. I was going to spoil her from day one. I even had a rocking chair to spend time rocking away the hours with her. I would have the time of my life with my lovely daughter. But, Heidi wasn't to be a baby in the baby sense. She was born a little adult. Her little eyes bounced around the house from day one. She was wide awake. That little girl was just days old, yet she was taking everything in. I was so amazed by this little wonder. She would cry when I put her in the crib and having been fed and changed. I couldn't figure out for the life of me what was the matter. I decided to look at the crib to see if there was anything in it that was disturbing her, and lo and behold, it was the bumper. She could not see out! So, I took it away and she stopped crying. This blew my mind. This baby was two weeks old and already she knew enough to realize that she could not see out, so she cried until I finally got it.

Heidi continued to stun me with her brilliance as a baby. Since I decided to breastfeed her, she had a 4 a.m. feeding and slept in her cradle at the foot of our bed. She would wake up on cue. I decided that four months was sufficient so I told her that she had to sleep all night and not wake up. Guess what? From that night on, she never woke up again. Heidi would sleep all night long. As I cleaned the house, I would place Heidi in her swing which played music and I would also put little books in the table part of the swing so she's have something to look at. Well, one day as I looked at her from the kitchen, she was turning the pages of the book. She was five months old. I could not believe my eyes. I said to myself, "Five months old and reading already." Every day was another surprise with her.

My husband Carl was the happiest man alive. He absolutely adored her. He strutted around like a peacock each and every day. I was so proud and happy with my little family. We had so much fun and I was so glad that I married Mr. Brandes. Heidi was too, the light of his life. He smiled all day long, nonstop. It was as though his cheeks were set in stone. He had a few business friends who would come to visit from time to time and just marvel at this miracle in his life. I kept thinking that it was the best decision I could have ever made.

I would set Huntington, New York ablaze with speculation, suspicion and subterfuge. The rumors would be rampant. How could this woman do this? Marry a man thirty-seven years her senior, and a white man at that. A young black teacher of a local, reputable and noted high school. What could she be thinking? It must be for his money. She couldn't possibly love him. Little did people know. Mr. Brandes and I already had a relationship. We were friends long before I moved into his house. I came to know him first as a printer. He had a business named Huntington Press. I was a patron. I had my extracurricular printing needs serviced by him. He was a sweet old man with a twinkle in his eye. His wife Eleanor died in 1979 and he was alone. When he told me this, I felt sorry for him and I offered to help him out. One day, he invited me over for dinner. I was stunned at how he was living. The house smelled like dogs. It was filthy, dark and reeked of death. It was like living in a tomb. My heart hit the floor. As I walked through the house, I realized that Mr. Brandes needed to be brought back to life and it was then that I decided he needed my help. I became his housekeeper. I took on the job of coming over and cleaning up the place after school and sometimes I would stay overnight when it was convenient. Afterwards, I decided to move to Huntington, and that's when Mr. Brandes offered me the upstairs apartment that he was building for his late wife's daughter and her children. But Mickey decided that she did not want to leave Florida since her kids were teenagers in high school. The apartment wouldn't be ready for a few more months, but it was going to be lovely. I was so excited.

In April of 1980, 655 Park Avenue in Huntington, New York became my new address. I was now a mile and a half away from my work. Life was good. I was leaving the hour long commute behind me as well as the tears and pain from Franklin Avenue.

Mr. Brandes and I got along so well. I did all the shopping, cooking and cleaning. I spent a lot of time downstairs with him to keep him from being lonely. We even started going out together. I took him to New York City to see a play. He invited me to the local bar. The Tuthill Lounge. It was run by a man named Royal who made the best chili in town. There was also a bartender named Nino whose favorite dish was pasta fagioli. We used to have so much fun in that little spot.

My family came to visit often and came to know Mr. Brandes quite well. My mother and father grew to be very fond of him. We were like family. That Thanksgiving and Christmas we all had dinner together downstairs with Mr. Brandes. It was one of the best times I ever had.

After the New Year, Mr. Brandes invited me downstairs for a special dinner. He asked me what I liked and I told him and he prepared everything I said. I was awestruck. He was also very well dressed. He had on a gleaming white lace shirt, gray trousers with creases that would slice a cake, shiny black shoes and his hair was slicked back flat on his head. He began to pace up and down in front of the fireplace ready to make what seemed like a speech. He stopped, turned, looked at me and said, "As you know, Helen, I am getting on in age and I do not have any family here. I would like you to consider this proposition. A proposition of marriage." My jaw dropped. He continued: "I know you are a young black woman who has to think about your reputation and what this would mean to you. And what people will say. This won't be easy." I am listening to this in utter amazement. All the while my mind is racing every which way. He ends with, "You, of course, would get the house, the building, and what money I have. You would be well provided for. Take your time and think this over, Helen. For you, this is a major decision." I said to myself, "You don't say!"

I went up to my apartment and said, "Wow! I don't believe this is happening." But it was. What was I to do? I decided to go away for the winter recess in February in New York City to think. There, I would do my own pacing back and forth. The one thing I knew for sure was that I could not leave Mr. Brandes. I realized that I cared for him. I liked him and, more importantly, he needed me. He relied and depended on me and that meant so much. But the question was, how could I do this and be happy, truly happy? I would have to have a baby. That was it. A child would make all the difference. I would finally be a mommy. I would have the one thing that I wanted of any marriage; my very own baby! I couldn't wait to get home to tell Mr. Brandes the good news. I was ecstatic and grinned from ear to ear. We decided to see his doctor to discuss the possibility of Carl fathering a child. His doctor said, "Of course he can be a father, go for it!" And so we did. Mr. Brandes asked me to move downstairs and I got pregnant the first time. I told Mr. Brandes that I wanted to get married on my birthday that coming August 15, 1981. We had a small wedding in his home. I invited my parents, sister, nieces, nephews, a few cousins and a few co-workers. Mr. Brandes smiled all day long and so did I.

It was a decision made out of fear. I had been in denial, real denial. My past had been filled with intense hurt, pain and disappointment. I was scared to death of my future. I was thirty years of age with no prospects of a future. I desperately wanted to have a child. Mr. Brandes would be safe. He would be the answer. Mr. Brandes would not deceive me, lie to me, hurt me in any way. He would be true. He would love me and need me. He was a Godsend. He would give me the one thing that I wanted and needed all my life: truth, honesty, loyalty, devotion and love. But more than anything else, I'd have a beautiful child. The child would not be dark skinned. The child would be light. This was important to me since I had been discriminated against. I was a "Little Darky." My child would never have this stigma. My child would be accepted for all for who she was and would be. My child would have a better chance at life and never experience the pain I felt as a young person of a darker hue. The thought of this made it worth everything. There would be nothing anyone could say about me in all this. My child would come first. The marriage would never be about money or material things.

I went on line today and there was an article about how and why so many people regain the weight they lose. The culprit is due to emotional eating. This is nothing new. Researchers have tagged this cause many times before, however, the problem remains. People are overcome by anxiety from loneliness and feelings of helplessness. These are often common characteristics in the battle against obesity. Scientists have yet to blend together both goals: the ability to lose the weight and the emotional counterpart to sustain the weight loss. Until then, for many of the millions who face this dilemma, there is no magic bullet.

As for myself, my battle is lodged in my past. My emotional self in a quagmire of confusion, self doubt, abandon, fear, despondency, distrust, isolation (self-imposed) and withdrawal. Spanning a lifetime based upon the occurrences and events that took place creating who and what I am today. Embedded in a system of beliefs punctuated by the realities and experiences lived. I have become stilted, stuck and strained to the point that I cannot surrender to anyone my deepest feeling, my heart, my soul. I am left guarded, vigilant and suspect of anyone who dares to tread into my safe haven. I let no one in, no one. I am my protector. I am my hero, my victor, my champion. I let no man enter this realm. I keep and will continue to keep all at bay. Accept God the Father, because, unlike man, God never goes back on His word. God is the only thing that I trust in life, He is all that I need. God is not a deceiver, a liar, an adulterer, a user, an abuser or a thief. I known all of those listed in my lifetime and I've had enough of these conditions which lead to "weight pain" and emotional eating.

My comrades who undergo continual yoyo dieting and binging only do so because they have yet to fill their hole, their pit, their cavern with their truths. The truths that are so painful, so devastating, so cruel. They need to dig down into the core of themselves and identify what's eating away at them. What's causing the weight pain? What's its root or roots? This must be figured out before real weight loss and maintenance can begin.

"Fat and skinny had a race, fat fell down and broke her face." It went something like this when I was a child. Did you ever hear such a thing during your lifetime? What was supposed to be the message? Were you to feel guilty about being fat? Were you to think that fat was bad? Whatever the intent, it was not good. We live in a society that never lets us forget that we were larger, chubbier, heftier, portlier, pudgier and wider than everyone else around us. We live in a society that punishes us for being rounder. It ignored us. It deleted us. It gave us tents to wear. It ridiculed us. It stared and jeered at us. It assaulted us. It swore at us. It made us crawl up and want to die.

Well, guess what? We're here to stay. Proud! Glorious! Wondrous! Hopeful! Beautiful! We are evolving into who we are and are meant to be. We, men and women alike are full of talent, intelligence, inspiration, creativity and genius. We are, too, the movers and shakers of the world. We are visionaries, pioneers, inventors and, above all else, we are investors who have a stake in this great land of ours.

Curves are in: look at Queen Latifah, Mónique, America Ferrera, Jennifer Hudson, Tyra Banks and Cameron Manheim. These ladies are all winners. They are changing the face and shape of Hollywood. Brava! The message is that we are not all destined to be the same. We are all unique in our own right. We are unique in our own skin, body type and frame. We decide what's best for us. This is our right and only ours to do. Remember, it's between you, your doctor and God! Leave it at that, you'll be better off.

For you guys out there, the same applies. The pressure is on you to have those abs, the washboard stomach. Now, is that realistic for you? Ask yourself, is this doable for me? If not, why make yourself crazy? Why dabble in steroids, if you have considered that route, which can be harmful to your health. Do what's convenient and easy for you. Simplify a workout routine three days a week. Something to give you a good cardiovascular workout. Check with your doctor for suggestions. Do a health care practitioner visit once a year for a full medical checkup. You guys don't do this often enough, which can prove critical to your health. Try to follow and practice healthy eating choices as mentioned. There hasn't been as much ballyhoo about you guys as there has been about women and size. Society has been more tolerant and accepting about big men. Maybe is goes back to the nineteenth century and the days of the robber barons, the big fat cats who controlled the major corporations in banking, steel and oil. In any event, guys get off a lot easier than women.

This isn't to say that men suffer in silence. Men have their moments of torment and self denial. Yes, we see only that which we want to see, since the reality is way too painful. We wear those blinders which obscure the whole or real picture of who we really are and look like. I have done this myself. I only see the imaginary size that I want to see until I walk past a store window and look at me, the real me. This hits home. I am forced to face my truth. Men are just as vulnerable as we are when it comes to weight issues. I think it's less emphasized, I think it's because we expect men to be stronger and I think it's because we as a society are more forgiving toward men because we see them as our providers, our protectors, our champions.

What's deep in the heart of a man? What bears down on his soul? Does he want to holler and scream like women do occasionally? I bet he does. Who's there for him in his weakest moment, when he's not full of triumph? When he sees himself as a failure? A lump? What keeps his head above water? Is his waist line a yardstick for his life's anxiety and pain? Is he too a victim of weight pain?

Our men bear the burden of the world on their shoulders daily. Their families, their jobs, their homes, the wars, the schools, the peace, the safety and more. They are overwhelmed. Constantly overwhelmed, pitted against good and evil, righteousness and indignation, rich and poor, and so much more. But, most of all, his desire to have a mate (her, too).

Emotional eating has several major dimensions: deprivation, loss, anxiety, happiness, emptiness, abandonment, depression, fear, lack of affection and rejection. Let me say that I am no clinician of any sort, by any means. I am merely stating what seems obvious to me, based upon my life experiences and observations. I have suffered through most, if not all, of these during my life at one time or another and still do. I will touch upon happiness since this may throw a curve by standing out. When I am very happy, based on something wonderful, a good turn of events, I eat. I eat as a reward. Does this sound familiar? I eat as a way of saying "Good job, well done." Or, "You deserve this." I thank myself. I show my appreciation to myself. Have you done this? Think about it. When things go wrong in our lives, we invariably resort to some destructive behavior. Overeating has become the culprit. Why? Because we can do it in silence, we can do it hidden, we can do it alone. It is our vice. It is our addiction. It is our nemesis. We feel helpless and out of control. We see the fat coming, but we can't stop it. We scream in silence. Our minds are consumed with food to erase away and diminish our pain. We can't escape. We can't elude it. It chases us down like a raging storm. We become numb with fullness, overdosed and clogged with food until the next fix. We're fighting a losing battle.

My daughter Heidi has become a victim of this syndrome which has been passed on by me. She was such a precious and precocious little girl. I failed her in the way that she needed me most. I was under the illusion that my little angel, being so brilliant, independent and self-sufficient, was okay on her own. I failed to realize that she still needed hugs, praises and kisses. I thought she was a little adult who didn't need me. She talked completely at thirteen months and walked at nine. I was always in awe of her development. I became her guardian, her protector and her provider. I gave her the best of everything that money could buy. She went to private schools, she went to gymnastics, she went to ballet school. She would have every advantage I could give her. I never had to help her with her homework. She got straight A's. I thought my role was to be a good role model, teach her how to be a good person with ethics, morality, good judgment and be successful in life. But, somehow, I missed the boat. Heidi had been deprived. She had not felt my love for her. She missed those hugs, those cuddles, those praises and those kisses. I left her with a hole in her gut, huge. She lacks portion control. She is still trying to fill the void that I left in her. She has been a little chubby, but lost the weight when she entered the Navy. She came down to 135 from 178. Heidi and I have talked about this and will work on it.

Be mindful, folks, this is a passed on tradition. The lack of tenderness is generational. As I said earlier, my parents never hugged and kissed me, either. Their parent's parents probably never did as well. We must stop this cycle. Children need all sorts of validation. Touching (good touching), hugging, kissing and saying "I love you" are the most important things a child needs for emotional well being. Along with praise and support. We don't do this enough. Parents today are pulled in so many directions, working two jobs in many cases don't have enough time to lavish their children with much needed love and attention. We all pay a price for this. We need to schedule family time every week to come together and have "huddle and hug parties" with the kids. Have old fashioned slumber parties in your rooms, parents. Invite the kids in, have pillow fights, watch old classic movies, eat popcorn, dress up in costumes, make it fun. The idea is never be too busy to play with your children! Also have family powwows. Clear out a space in the living room or family room, sit in a circle and have talks about what's going on in the world today, or in their school community, neighborhood, with them and keep those lines of communication open. For younger children, play ball toss or card games and the reward should always be higs and kisses. Play happy music and dance together. My children and I used to go outside when it rained and danced around on warm summer days. They lost so many pairs of shoes down the drain. But it was fun. The bottom line is: folks, be mindful of your children's emotional health because someday it may haunt them.

We let our world swallow us up whole, spitting out the pit and the core of our most delicious fruit. We abandoned out senses for a pound of fat. We left our senses out in the trenches cold, damp, shivering relentlessly. We dug ourselves into a hole and never stopped filling it up. We were looking for safety and comfort from the outside elements and it never came.

So here we are, a product of the environment. We are confused, tormented, disgusted, outraged, aggravated, sorrowful, pitiful and obese.

Our families, God love them. They did their best to console us as children.

They wiped those little tears away when you got a booboo. They hugged you (some of you) when you needed it. They gave you something to make you FEEL better. Bingo! This is implanted deeply, down in your subconscious. These memories are the crux of your eating pattern. You want to release the hurt and the pain. You want to soothe, stroke, comfort, heal and "make" you feel better. Just like your mommy did. Since what she gave you to eat tasted so yummy, so tasty and was so timely. You began to learn and identify when to do this during your lifetime, and you never stopped.

You were also told to "Eat everything on your plate. Don't you know that there are starving kids out there who would kill for that food?" We have all heard this at some point of another. So you cleaned your plate even though it meant stuffing yourself and you eventually got used to it. There was no such thing as portion control back in the day. Sounds like something from outer space, right? But it's the buzz phrase of the day. Restaurants did away with averaging portions in order to compete. It's a tough business. So, the wise among them devised this concept of "family style" which not only was like home cooking, but huge portions as well. A whole new phase of eating out was born. "Supersize me!" says McDonald's and a "weigh" we go!

You can see fat coming, it doesn't sneak up on you. But many of us choose to either ignore it or simply let it happen. We don't know why. It just keeps coming and we walk around oblivious to the person who we are becoming. I am saying "we" because I have done this also. We can't seem to help ourselves; we wouldn't know why, but when we look into our mirrors we see a distortion of ourselves.

The image we see in that mirror is plain, pure and simple. It's a vast complexity of our inner psyche. It's a vast enigma and chasm that lurks all around us, through us, deep within. We are helpless. Food has become our provider. It has become the deliverer. It has become the source of our self hatred. This is powerful. This is mind blowing.

We live in a world that caters to our senses. The visual is the most profound, the most sensual, the demanding, if you will. What you see is what you think you want and what you think you want is what you get. You don't have a choice. You have to belong, you have to be part of the crowd, you have to be accepted, no matter what. You lack the discipline to say no. You lack the will to say no, even to yourself. Our society rules every waking moment of our lives and you don't realize it. You don't know that there are signals impairing your judgment. I used to think about the absence of chubby people, average looking people, physically challenged people on TV and in advertisements when I was growing up. They were hidden. They were left out. They were outcast. They were the ones who nobody wanted. We were programmed to only accept beauty in all forms. Even skin color was an issue. Light skin was far more desirable than dark. Long hair was far more desirable than short. Blonde hair was more the rave than red. Systematically, we were bombarded and hoodwinked. We looked at ourselves and said "Yeech!" So we ate away our undesirability. We ate away our brilliance. We ate away our beauty and settled for mediocrity.

People do not understand the 2% of you who keep it off. Bravo. The other 98% is still in lockdown. Your emotional self, your trauma self, if you will, is directly related to both size and degree of ills. One of the hardest things to do in this life is to live with other people! Family, friends, co-workers, etc., etc. It's all the same, no difference. You need to seek out in you, in your heart and in your mind, who hurt me? Who rejected me? Who stabbed me in my heart in my life's experience? What pain did I encounter? Can I forgive? Can I release? Can I let go?

You have to dig and dig.

If not, weight loss will not be possible, sustainable or manageable. Lest we not forget, the emotional eating that is part and parcel to this cycle and repetition. Eating for reward, happiness, fear, loneliness, etc., etc. All of this is part of the invisible core self. These are your unseen, your hidden arena in which you constantly battle the demons within yourself.

Real weight loss takes time, conscious time, in your present state of mind. There's nothing quick about it. It's a long-term process. You are an architect. You are its planner. You are its advisor. You are the benefactor. Do not participate in the get rich quick scheme for all the diet companies. You are their mark, their profit target, you are being scammed over and over again. Why do you think you became a compulsive eater, an anorexic, a bulimic? Pain and more weight pain made you this way. Society and its "skinny" compulsive excessive behavior made you crazy and out of control. Did you ever stop to think about people who lived thousands of years ago? Do you think they went through this nonsense? Hell, no! Beauty was manifested in myriad ways: scarifications, size, beauty adornments, tattoos, etc. Think about it. There have been fat people, big people, large people, obese people throughout mankind's history. It's only in the 20th century that this weight trauma syndrome began. Why? Because there's MONEY in it! Wake up people. Back in the days, cowboys slept with as many big women as they did small. Do you think they cared after being on a trail drive for four to six months what size she was and wanted to get some? No, they snatched the first thing they saw. And pumped up until they both exploded. Think about Rubens. His portraits were of chubby women. Statues of African art included chubby women.

Go do your homework. We were fat and happy back in the day folks! Think about all the problems we have today in this lifeeverything boils down and reduces to MONEY. We are systematically bred to be fat. Then we are forced into the guilt of being fat, then made to lose the weight while the big fat cats make billions from our fat little backs. Don't continue giving these companies the satisfaction.

Take charge of your own destiny!

Dieting has become America's favorite pastime.

Count the food commercials on TV. They are numerous, then here come the diet commercials. You are on a revolving door spiral. Do you really think anyone wants you to lose weight? The major drug and diet companies? Hell, no!

If we don't stay fat, they don't make money. And who's laughing all the way to the bank?

We are all guinea pigs for the rich. Why do you think they separate themselves from us? Yeah, they live in their own world and talk about us, like dogs, behind our backs. They keep us poor. They keep us struggling. They keep us anxious. They keep so many of us in the ghetto, planned communities, so we can get sick, so they can come to our rescue. We are fed subliminal messages daily with all the gusto they can muster. We are talking about some of the most powerful families and companies today. Believe me, I don't want to piss these guys off. They are roguish, ruthless and relentless! Fellow Americans, take charge of yourselves and your bodies. Live for yourselves.

September 26, 2002 would be a day to change my life for the rest of my days. I would have a terrible car accident and never return to work again. I would on that day bid Huntington High School adieu. My colleagues, my students, my memories would be forever entwined in the corridors of one of them most important edifices of my entire life. I spent most of my adult life in those hallowed halls. I loved every minute of it. It was the most wondrous working experience of my entire life. I can't go into everything that took place there; that's another book. I will always smile when I think of my life and times there. Including the pounds I gained and lost during my trials and tribulations. Yet, many days brought pain and anguish from those who crossed the barriers of human kindness, goodwill, love, patience, sympathy, caring, sharing and all that which warms and calms the spirit and the soul. Huntington High School kept me grounded and, on many occasions, kept me sane. There would be days when I would leave home and slam the car door and say to myself, "this is my sanctuary, my peace." And so it was. Even with all that was going on in my building during my latter years after my father died in 2002, my move back to Brooklyn, my ailing mother, my son's depression, I was on a mission to survive. Huntington held me up. My dear friend Camille held me up. She was the school librarian. Caring, intelligent, stoic, dedicated to her profession and the voice of reason. She was my sounding board. She was my confidant. She was my soul sister. We were joined at the hip. I needed to see her face every day. Without it, I fought the demons within me, with my depression raging; I battled with my weight.

Up and down the scales I climbed. The weight pain was a merry-go-round. I would come to work every day as though all was good in my life and nothing was further from the truth. My life was a living Hell. Before we left Huntington, my son was getting more and more depressed. The atmosphere did not help. He met kids who enticed him to cut out and I was the Dean of Students. He had a fight in the gym, claiming he was defending the honor of another. Two days later, I would hear over the radio, "Mrs. Weeks, Christopher left the building." If knew that if I was to manage I had to leave Huntington and moving to Brooklyn would be the answer.

No it wasn't and Christopher had a meltdown.

Brooklyn turned out to be a disaster. I knew that we had to get out of there. It wasn't just the drugs, but also the safety issue. My father as well as my brother were both mugged on those mean streets and I began fearing for my son. Christopher, in his despair and loneliness for Long Island, wanted to travel back and forth to see his friends. One night I had to wait up until 3:30 a.m., until he came home. Every horrible scenario ran through my mind and it became clear to me that he must have a car. Off I went to a Jeep dealership and bought a used Jeep Grand Cherokee with everything in it to keep my son safe, even though he'd be driving only with a leaner's permit. I didn't care. I would take full responsibility. The worry and anxiety over Christopher's well being stabilized and so did my waistline.

Families of America, you have the hardest task of all. Feeding yourselves. But, I have a few suggestions for you as well. First, curtail fast food dining. Yes, I know it's fast and convenient and tastes good too, however, pounds, pounds, pounds and more pounds add up over time. Do you think this is nutritious or healthy, especially for the kids? How about the mother who tried suing McDonald's for making her child fat? This was one of the most insane things I have ever heard. You have the full responsibility of deciding what to put into your children's little mouths. Second, cook with the kids. Make them part of meal planning and preparation. When my son was a little boy, he loved to cook with me. He would say, "Mom, don't start without me." Today, he's a cook and someday wants to own a restaurant now that he has completed his course of study at the Scottsdale Culinary Institute here in Arizona. Who cares if you wreck the kitchen? Have the kids help you clean up. Start this process when they are between three and five. Working moms, pick a day of the week when you can cook with the kids and freeze what you make. Family meal planning is essential today. Dads as well can participate in this endeavor. Go to bookstores and read through books and copy out recipes and try them. Third, teach the kids to make their own lunch for school. On TV, you always have mom making lunch. Let them do it. All you need to do is stand by and help with the cutting, if necessary. This will give them a sense of added purpose. Hopefully, they won't toss the lunch because they made it.

Obesity in children, with the exception of medical reasons, is appalling. On the "Maury' show, mothers have brought in their toddlers, weighing in at over 100 pounds! Their rationale is "He cries!" or "He throws a tantrum if I don't give it to him!" Lady, are you crazy, or what? This is enabling, destructive, abhorrent behavior on the part of the parent or parents. This is leading a child to a slow and miserable death. My question is: where are the other family protestations? As I said earlier, you see fat coming. It doesn't just sneak up on you.

Families, please beware. Feed your children with love and sense.

Another critical concern I have is for those who are literally shut in because they are too large, too huge, too obese to move out of their homes. Remember a man named "Tiny," a black man who was shut in his home due to excessive obesity? He made the headlines some years ago and has since died. Well, he could not move. He was planted in his bedroom, weighing more than I can remember. The point that I am making here is how did Tiny get that way? He had help. His family, with their misplaced love, helped to feed himself to death. They gave him everything he wanted to eat. People, please, please, please don't said in this horrible death trap. Get help immediately for your loved ones. Why should the fire department have to come and cut a hole in the side of the house to extricate them? There are probably countless others hidden amongst us. If you know of anyone, talk to their families and urge them to get help. There's no shame here, folks. You are saving a life!

I am a baby boomer and I don't remember this phenomenon. I dined out quite a bit when I lived in New York City. I ate out in the East Village, Chinatown, Little Italy. Columbus Avenue in the 70's, Restaurant Row (Midtown). Portions were, top me, average back then. If you lived in Brooklyn, like I did, it was Junior's on Flatbush Avenue that was the place to go. You got the "nosh" goodies on the table, sour dill pickles, cole slaw and pickled beets.

Our society consumes us with food every waking hour. You can't get away from it. You can even drive up to food from your vehicle. Burger King, Wendy's, McDonald's are all addicting. You can drive up and order enough food for three or four people, go home or park somewhere and eat it all yourself. Sound familiar? And every bite you take is a hurt, pain, rejection, crisis, event, torment, fear and worry that have been emblazoned in your heart of hearts. Every bite is a cry for help. Every bite is not about the FOOD. Instead of eating the food, you need to ask yourself, "What's eating YOU?" Before you binge, before you overeat, before you clean that plate, ask yourself "What am I running from? What am I afraid of? Who hurt me? What am I ashamed about? What are my hidden fears? Why do I think I am not good enough? What do I really want out of LIFE?" In other words, search your soul, look inside, deep inside. Don't be fearful of facing these demons. Clean out your house, clear your head once and for all. Your life depends on it. What you look like, what you really think, what you really believe in, your inner core self is between you, your doctor and God.

If you have major health issues, the same is true.

Get help! Seek out meaningful relationships with reliable and trustworthy people. Where do you find them? In your place of worship, Overeaters Anonymous, hotlines and community groups. You need non-judgmental feedback and constant support. Think of it as a withdrawal from a condition. It is. It will be a re-conditioning, a slow and gradual process of evolution. It will be cathartic, a metamorphosis, a therapeutic re-awakening. An emergence of a new wholesome self. More alive, more vibrant and more confidant. There'll be no stopping you. The cocoon will be shed. It will be like being re-born. Your state of happiness will soar. You will learn what real and true happiness means. The chains and shackles that enslaved your mind will disappear forever. Are you feeling this? Can you visualize this? Want it! See yourself in your mind's eye the way you truly want to be. You can be your dream. You can be your desire. You can be your hope. Do not leave this to anyone else but you. You have the ability to be. Release it.

Cleanse your body as well as your mind. Enlighten yourself spiritually. Come out fighting. You have to learn to look at this world and say "I'm here in the 'me' that 'I' am." In the me that I love. In the me that I cherish. In the me that I adore. Inspired, hopeful, encouraged and ready to live your best life.

Book II

Practical Wisdom for Weight Maintenance

Introduction

Have you ever been up and down the scale? Have you been "queen" or "king" of the "Yoyo" Syndrome? Sure, we all have. But, now, it's time to look at simple ways to manage and keep your weight down and at your desired level. No tricks, no fads, no gimmicks, just plain common sense and easy ways that can make all the difference in how you look and feel are described herein. All you need in an open mind and a willingness to adopt these suggestions. No matter what you've lost here are 50 ways to keep you where you want to be. Studies show that over 90% of all people who lose weight gain it back and more. I'm sure many of you dieters know the agony of this behavior and can't, for the life of you, figure out why this is happening.

This guide is really about a "new" relationship that you're going to have with yourself. After all, who is the one who needs to benefit from all of your past efforts? That's right! You are! So now, all you need to do is take a closer look at how you manage your daily habits and behavior to help control and maintain your weight. There's really no need to struggle day after day to keep an "imaginary" ideal weight. This means a societal and self-imposed image of what you "think" you must look like. This is not realistic and only causes stress, depression and anxietyfor you as well as most other people. We live in a society that constantly bombards us with the need to lose weight for our overall health. This is true. If we are subject to those dreaded diseases, diabetes, high blood pressure, and the rest of those ailments that plague us, imprison our hopes, our spirit, and drain our energy; we need a remedy. But fear not. Stop and think.

Ask yourself: what weight range can I live within? What weight range can help me feel comfortable with me? What weight range is realistic for me? Is my weight range three to five pounds? Five to ten pounds? Is this something that I can monitor? Realistically? Whatever you decide is RIGHT for you. Yet, your doctor will assuredly insert his or her own input, and that's okay, depending on your individual state of health. Keep in mind that this is a totally "new relationship" that you are embarking on with yourself. There was an old commercial in the 1980s that said, "There's a new you coming every day." Make this your mantra, your affirmation, hold onto those words. They inspire, incite and encourage. Rid yourself of the doubt that you cannot do this. Yes, you can. No matter what size you are, no matter how you look, no matter what anyone else thinks. This is about you. So, here it is. Let's get rolling!

1. Get a hobby! Find a hobby! What do you like to do in your spare time? Are you good with your hands? Can you make or build something? What creative talent or ability lurks within you? Tap into your innermost reaches and yank something out. Knitting, sewing, drawing, sketching? What is your heart's desire? Find it! Do it! Release your inner genius! We all have it! This will help to balance as well as soothe the nervous energy in your core self. Diminishing the desire to eat out of control needs channeling. Busying your hands as well as your mind is essential for weight maintenance.

2. Get a full-length mirror. Do not hide from yourself. See what others see and work at accepting it. This is an everyday process. Your feelings about your physical self will be tested. So start facing it. Oh, by the way, you married folks and partners are just as involved in this endeavor. You will need to be a helper, not a hindrance (so check yourselves, too).

3. Rearrange your closets, drawers and shelves. Make yourself "work" for what you need to find in your home. Every form of movement helps. So, start with your immediate environment, not just parking your car a block or two away.

4. Plan to eat one "good" meal a day. I will discuss this more later on. We all like to have our favorite foods; this is a given. Pick

the meal in your day that you most want to enjoy and savor. Whether it's breakfast, lunch or dinner, it is not important. The idea is that you can't and shouldn't indulge yourself at every meal. For example, if breakfast is a favorite of yours, make three of your favorite things to eat. For example, most of us like eggs, bacon, sausage, toast, French toast, pancakes (my sister loves hominy grits), whatever. Pick them! That is your food focus for the day! Enjoy whatever you have selected. Prepare them just the way you like, but take your time eating. This meal should last at least fifteen to twenty minutes. In doing so, you savor every bite, every smell, aroma and flavor. The idea is to make this meal into a ceremony. A fete! Taste everything. We are gobblers when we eat. The thing here is sensual. Yes, sensual! Make it a ritual. Why? Because you like to eat. In doing this, you can eat without the guilt afterward, as many of us to when we binge, stuff ourselves and gorge while eating. But there is a catch. Once you do this, you are finished eating like this for the day. This means that the other two meals let are just plain and simple. You are, however, still eating what you want. Let's be clear about this. The meal you savored and enjoyed was the most special, the most sublime. You had everything that you wanted, so not the other meals will be moderately consumed with wholesome choices. I mean healthier, leaner, fat-free or low-fat. You get the idea. Oh, and portions, portions, portions, portions, please work at managing these over time.

5. Add more fresh fruit to your eating choices. Eat more of what's in season. Many people do not think to add fruit to any meal. Start! I eat fruit not only with breakfast, but with lunch and dinner, too. Instead of eating a green salad, why not make it a fruit salad? If you remember going to a catered affair, what's the first thing you eat? Fruit! A fruit cup. This gets all the digestive enzymes ready for what's coming next. The good stuff, right?

6. Change the time of day you eat the biggest meal. When I traveled to Barbados to see my relatives, the biggest meal was noontime. Boy did we eat! Meats, rice, potatoes and dessert. But the evening was totally calmer. You ate light. Small snacks like a few slices of fruit, cheese, maybe a slice of what we call

deli meat, bread (though not a sandwich) and drinks made with rum. It was the same in Germany with my husband's family. Dinner was early, at 4:00 p.m., and awesome. Meat, lots of potatoes and carrots which are big over there, salad and beer. At about 8:00 or 9:00 p.m., you had similarly what was typical. Bread with butter and slices of the leftover meat, if there was any left over. This was quite a few years ago, but I will never forget how people outside the United States eat. Try to keep night time eating light. This is a problem for many people. At night, the harried day is laid to rest, we get the nibbles, munchies or whatever you want to call it. I suggest making a trail mix for those moments. I do. Start with a favorite cereal, like Wheat Chex ® which comes in three types. Pick one, then you can add nuts, pretzels, dried fruit, raisings, etc. This stuff hits the spot. Whatever you decide, try not to eat anything considered "heavy" at night, especially after 8:00 p.m.

7. Develop your inner spiritual self. I am not advocating that you become a nun or monk. I am asking you to look inward a little more often. You ask how? Meditate. If you do not know how, just start sitting quietly for about ten minutes. Most people cannot do this any longer. In this time, simply let your mind be quiet. Focus on your breathing. Inhale, exhale. Take breaths in and let them out slowly. If you'd like to count to a number, then do so. Work at this. It may feel strange at first, but you'll come to like it and feel refreshed. You can also sit and listen to soothing music. Something instrumental perhaps? Experiment with this. I like Native American songs.

8. Find a toddler(s) to baby sit once in awhile. These little kids three to five years of age are not only energetic, but are fun to be with. They make you laugh, keep you moving (chasing after them) and they remind you how to have innocent fun which is good for your spirit. You will also get exercise and be reminded that you are never too old to play.

9. Walk an elderly person or someone in your family around the neighborhood. You get to walk slowly and have a conversation at the same time. I love the elderly, they are full of stories about the past and are walking history lessons. Many of them are so

eager to share with younger people. Seek them out for their comfort as well as your own.

10. Make new friends. Talk to people. Anywhere. Strike up a conversation. In line at the store, at your bank, on the street corner. Why? Because you need to come out and feel validated. Yes, you need to be heard as well as recognized in your skin! You need to let people know that you have something to say. It doesn't have to be a dissertation or a blueprint for a skyscraper. You just want to be acknowledged, if only for a moment. In doing that, you are beginning to accept the "body in tow." Yours. Some of you, the "chubbettes" (this is my term for the chubby amongst us). I dislike the word obese. Yuk! It carries such negativity. You are not negative. You are buds waiting to blossom into your unique selves and you may be shy, a little introverted and have been unassuming. So, speak up. A little at a time until you become more comfortable with yourself. You are not to be hidden within. You matter.

11. Learn a new sport or a new game. Find people in your community to interact with. Your place of worship is a good place to start. Bingo anyone? Keeping busy is imperative to staying on course. The idea is to fill your sphere of activities. Get off that computer! Slow down on the chat rooms. Stop being a chat room junky. That only allows for hiding from direct face to face contact and it is too impersonal (this is one woman's opinion). I enjoy the real thing. You should too. Remember people are everywhere. So, get out! Be seen! Smile!

12. Hang a different dress of shirt on your door every day. This is to remind you of your own versatility, changeability, adaptability and flexibility as a person. This is a practice in spontaneity and the chameleon aspects of your personality. You need to know what you can experience (all the things that come into your life). Your life is like your wardrobe. It can be spicy, alluring, practical, bold, daring, intense, flavorful. It can also be dull or boring. The point is, to show yourself the person you can be or want to be. All it takes is awareness. What better way is there to see you. Unless what you hang up is a reflection of

who you THINK you are. Then if you don't like what you see, a change has got to come. Get a new wardrobe. Do you have anything sexy?

13. Write! Get rid of stress, worry, tension, etc. Talk to yourself on paper. Be your own good listener. Be honest with yourself. Get it all out. Whatever it is that keeps you motionless, among the dead, among the dearly departed, put on paper! Bring yourself back to the living. Awaken refreshed, regenerated and raring to go. Break free on paper. Dig it out of your subconscious. The albatross around your neck that you've been carrying around all your life. Face those demons. When you're done, BURN IT! Whew! It's all gone!

14. Be your own cheerleader. Who better than you to root, to cheer and rah rah rah for you than you? Why leave this for someone else? You are so busy being your own worst enemy criticizing, belittling and beating yourself up. So, why can't you be your own number one supporter? You're one of the best friends you'll ever have, right? Right! Well?

15. Go to the beaches, parks, mountains, anywhere in Nature. Commune with open spaces, breathe in fresh air and even go for a walk in the rain on warm days. You have no idea how uplifting and joyous this can be. Consume your environment. No matter whether it is urban, suburban or rural, there is your own place in the sun. Feed your spirit. Remember the scene in *Pretty Woman* in which Richard Gere took off his shoes and when walking in the grass barefoot? If you saw the movie, try remembering the expression on his face. Think about it.

16. I listen to good soothing music. Gospel, opera, instrumentals. You can go to Borders and listen free. Listen to music in your head. I hum to myself or sing in my head. My grandmother hummed all the time, so I guess I picked it up from her.

17. Try new foods. Experiment. Browse through ethnic cookbooks. Again, go to Borders or any other bookstore and write down new menus. You get so stuck on what mama cooked and this becomes your mainstay. I'm sure she wouldn't mind if you

ventured out just a little to seek out other salubrious foods that you might find interesting.

18. By the way, make going to bookstores a regular part of your entertainment world. Fascinating things happen at book stores. Lectures, book signings, people watching, being seeing and these are just a few.

19. Pamper yourself once a month (men as well as women). Get that facial, pedicure, manicure you keep putting off because you think you'll feel silly or you may be embarrassed about the way you look. That's the point! Get a makeover, buy some new clothes. Excess poundage does not mean that you stop living. Hello! You are attractive, beautiful and resplendent no matter what size you are. You are worth it!

20. Keep your interest up. Keep yourself intellectually stimulated. Read the newspaper, or more than one if you have the resources, then throw in magazines and community newsletters. In other words, don't let dust collect in your brain. Remember, since you are getting out and interacting more, you need more stuff to talk about.

21. Invite people more often than you have. Don't fret about what your home looks like. Real friends don't really care. Play games. I love Po-ke-no and bingo (I am the Bingo Caller at the Queen Creek Senior Center in Queen Creek, Arizona.). Have everyone bring low calorie snacks and treats.

22. Join a recipe club or start your own. You can easily do this on line. The emphasis should be on low carbohydrate, low calorie meals. This can work with co workers and church people as well.

23. Find a walking partner at work and stroll around at lunchtime. You don't want to work up a sweat. Just take a relaxing stroll around the building or grounds three or four times a week. By the way, while you sit at your desk or work station, tap your feet and bounce your legs. Keep that body in motion!

24. Sleep in sexier clothes. Throw away anything flannel unless you live in the arctic. Sleep in sexy nighties, black lace (it comes in plus sizes), pastels, animal patterns and see through negligees. All systems go! You ain't dead yet! And guys, no matter what size you are, there's something to be said for a bare chest.

25. Be creative. Start a journal. Keep track of all the new and exciting experiences. Anything that puts a smile on your face is worth recording, after all, you have already burned in the bad stuff.

26. Start a club. Keep it small. Why? You need a support system. You need to be with people who share similar concerns and issues. Men and women alike should nestle themselves along with three to five others who will keep one another grounded. Agree to keep all matters private and confidential among yourselves. Trust and loyalty are paramount. You need to feel secure, protected, loved and respected by one another. This is a necessary ingredient for weight maintenance. This will help diminish the need for binge eating when alone. Keep a regular schedule for when you should meet. Plan activities that you all enjoy. Incorporate field trips out in Nature, menu planning and food shopping together and most of all, lots of hugs, embraces and touching when you are together. Remember, each of you is special and you should treat each other accordingly. This is the best way to express your sharing and caring. Don't forget to come up with a name for your club.

27. This one is hard, especially if you are partnered with someone else. Get rid of the TV in the bedroom. Do you realize how much snacking goes on in the bedroom? Some people even have little refrigerators in their bedrooms. For me, this is a no no. I do not have a TV in my bedroom. Think of your bedroom as a sanctuary, a place for rest, restoration and relaxation. It should be the one room in the house that is freed of and exempt from the troubles of the outside world. It should be your haven, your comfort zone, your paradise, if you will. My bedroom is my most favorite room in my house. It is where I commune with God. It is where I dream, visualize, where I

conjure up the spirit within me. It is my HOME away from my home. I love my bedroom. It is also where my inspiration and ideas are manifested. When I first awaken in the morning, I say "Hello!" and "Good Morning!" to God. We may even have a dialogue with me, of course, doing all the talking. I also look out the window and look at the sky. I love the sky. Here in Arizona, the mornings are beautiful, wondrous and invigorating. I also look for the birds that chirp and flit around. I absolutely love the peace and serenity that my bedroom brings me. Wallow in your bed. Get fluffy pillows, lots of pillows with bright bold colors, shades, hues. Soft sheets feel good on the skin (Remember no flannel bedclothes!). Make up your bed every day. Even if you just throw the covers up, it is enough. Also, no clothing on the floor. Keep this space tidy. No matter what you look like, bask in the glory of you in your bedroom. It is the first room you see, the first images of the day, the first sounds in and out of your mind. It provides for the first steps in your day which can set the pace, the mood and mental images of the day you may be apt to encounter. I can hear the mommies of the world screaming "Who are you kidding? I have three kids that I have to jump out of bed for every morning!" Even so, you should rethink what your bedroom should be. And there is one paramount rule: NEVER FIGHT IN THE BEDROOM.

28. Devise an AEP. This is an Alternate Eating Plan. Learn how to substitute foods and eating patterns. For example, when I know that I am going to travel, the few days before, I eat sparingly. I eat lots of fresh fruit, cereals and salads. Why? So I can eat what I want when I am on vacation and not feel guilty. I lose at least three to five pounds before I travel. This is so I can look forward to all the new and exciting foods I will eat, most of which I probably do not cook at home. In this way, you can accomplish several goals at once. One, you can minimize weight gain while you travel, and not space out at the thought of food. Next, put food (meals) on a schedule as you would any other appointment. Plan to eat that steak, rack of ribs, mashed potatoes with gravy and those smothered pork chops on a calendar planner. I eat steak two to three times a year, spare ribs two to four times a year, fried chicken one or

two times a year. Are you getting this? I think it is fun to plan the "Ritual of Eating" in this manner. You have something fun to look forward to, just like your holidays. For your birthday, a special favorite meal should be planned. This gives you not only the satisfaction of enjoying something yummy, it provides the anticipation of it coming. Book your favorite meals in advance. Even make one special thing a month, pick a "favorite food day." Caution! This does not mean that you pig out, all it means is that you are not restricting or omitting your favorites from your menu choices. The bottom line is to undo years of improper eating habits and food choices which made you grow around the waist in the first place. The one thing or feeling that people want to eliminate is desperation, denial and deprivation. This is perhaps why most, if not all, diets fail.

29. Eat more OATMEAL! Remember when you were a kid and your mother or grandmother made you eat that hot, steaming bowl of oatmeal? My grandmother, whom I am named after, made my sister and me farina, Wheatena® and oatmeal. She made it so sweet with sweetened, condensed milk which still makes my mouth water when I think of those times. You can even make one of those favorites at night for a snack, especially in the wintertime. By the way, these cereals are low fat, cholesterol free and low sodium. You can even top them with fruit or fruit preserves.

30. Add more steps to your daily routine and life. Keep that body in motion. Seek out what kind of devices you can use while sitting, standing or leaning to create body movement. Earlier, I suggested to bounce and tap your feet under your desk at work. Find one of those squeeze, hand held items to use; ten minute intervals will do nicely. This is a bit extreme, but I do it when I visit someone's home. I find things to clean. I visited my cousin in Henderson, Nevada and one morning, as everyone slept, I vacuumed the hallway, cleaned the kitchen counter and swept the kitchen floor. This took about a half an hour, but I worked up a sweat and I felt great. When one of my younger cousins inquired about my overzealous behavior I just said that this was my way of keeping my body in motion. It was my way of

getting some exercise. Then she quickly said, "Well, the floor needs washing!" And I smiled, but I did not clean the floor. I also clean up my neighborhood. I am one of the few people on my street who does not work, so I occasionally go to my neighbors' yards and do the weeding or water their plants. The house next to me is not yet occupied, so I water and prune the front yard, as well as the back. This not only keeps me busy, but I also get to be outdoors, in the sun, doing something I truly enjoy. For you city dwellers, pound that pavement. Walk, go sightseeing, window shop, go to parks, museums and take it all in. Absorb every eye opening, eye popping, eye stopping event. Savor and take delight in your city's grandeur. Rekindle, revive and regain the freshness that your environment offers. For the most part, it's all free, too! Go to your city centers, your town hall, your library, even go back to your old school. Keep yourself mentally stimulated, visually as well as aesthetically. My dearly departed Aunt Cheryl lived in New York City. She was not a well or wealthy woman, but she walked all over New York City. She knew Central Park like the back of her hand. She was exceedingly spiritual. Cheryl loved Nature. She loved being out there. Expand your horizons. Open those vistas and you won't have time to add on weight. You will be so busy with life that the over consumption of food will gradually disappear. You'll have to find the time to eat.

31. Smile and laugh more. Isn't laughter the best medicine? There's an old saying (I don't know where it came from) that you can laugh your way to health. So, why not laugh your way to weight stabilization? Look for humor all around you. There's some funny stuff going on out there. I don't mean cruel or malicious stuff. I mean fun stuff. I love to observe little kids. They do the funniest things. I once watched a little three year old put his sandals on the wrong feet and when he got up to walk away, he waddled like a duck. I laughed until I almost cried. I also love children's hairstyles, especially the do-it-yourself ones. You can always tell when they do. The hair is piled up on top of their heads in a lopsided hair clip, of they're wearing the sweep look in which all the hair is pushed to one side and, of course, no comb or brush was used. Better yet, you'll know when they dressed themselves: nothing matches.

Find things out there that put a smile on your face. When I go out sometimes, I plan on smiling at three (or more) people, complimenting them in the process. I especially pay attention to the "chubby" among us. We do need to validate one another. Tell him or her that they look nice. If it's a guy and his hair looks nice, tell him. If it's a gal wearing a nice outfit, tell her. I am an usher and greeter at my church where I stand in the front lobby before the first service at 9:00 a.m. and I make it a point to compliment at least five people every Sunday. "What a beautiful outfit!" or "You look lovely today!" or "I like that blouse, how pretty you look today!" I also hug people in all sizes and shapes. You cannot know how such a seemingly small gesture can make someone's day! Notice people around you, pay compliments and, one day, it will be your turn to receive them.

32. Keep an open mind as well as a sense of humor. Become more fun. Lighten up. Kick the doldrums to the curb. I am not telling you to change your personality, all I am saying is to be more open to fun and amusement. If you are a member of the "powder head set" (you have gray hair), you will still want to be fun and exciting to be around. As we age and watch our families and friends move on, it can depress you. Stay connected to people. Get out! Have fun! It's good for your well-being and self image. Keep negative people far, far away. Think of that as a plague you do not want to catch.

33. Come out into the open. Don't hide or shut yourself up in your home. Don't cocoon yourself out of the way of fear. Participate in local activities. Go to the auto show. Or the home show. Maybe the flower show. Lectures and seminars are available out there. Seniors get in for half price at most of these events. Also go to your state fair, if you live nearby. Keep active! Also, listen to the sounds around you. Occupy your thought with things that are positive. Bring your physical and environmental world in. Notice the beauty that surrounds you. The trees, flowers, scents, aromas, birds, small animals and creatures. Consume your environment every day. Notice the subtleties, the movement around you, especially the colors. Colors are essential and very soothing as well as stimulating. Look up at

the sky. See the baby blue hues. The snow white caps and the shady gray clouds. This is awesome! As you look up and gaze, wish, dream, hope, imagine, wonder, visualize and create positive thoughts. This is good for your blood pressure.

34. Go dancing or take dancing lessons. One of the biggest crazes now is just that. Since "Dancing with the Stars" aired, membership in dance clubs and ballrooms has soared. If you don't want to go out in public, then sponsor a dance night in your home. Have dance parties. Salsa, rumba, cha cha, tango, Lindy Hop, do the slop (this is really old school) do your heart's content.

35. Het a new "do." Het a hair makeover. Shorten it. Lengthen it. Bob it. Perm it. Color it. Guys can grow a mustache, beard, goatee or whatever. Take the plunge! Don't be afraid to change. Change happens every day, whether you realize it or not.

36. Fill your world with beauty, surround yourself with plants and flowers. They bring peace, comfort, love and joy. Touch them. Talk to them. Nurture them. Water them. Say good morning and good night to them. They will thrive in the spirit of your gentleness and kindness.

37. Accept the new look you have acquired. Smile at yourself in the mirror on a daily basis.

38. Accept the way you appear to others. This is not your problem. It's theirs. My stomach hangs. So what? Two babies, belly rolls and flab give me added character.

39. Become more mysterious. Get people guessing about the new you. They will want to know what is going on. Add intrigue! Add spice! Become unpredictable. Become more spontaneous! Remember, there is a new you coming every day.

40. Get rid of your fears about your size. Come to terms with it. Some chubby people have a phobia about public transportation. That seat is not quite big enough, and they spill over into the next seat. You have a choice: you can either

sit or stand. I don't recommend that you sit or stand for ten to thirty minutes en route to your destination. Sit down. The seat you leave behind will accommodate a child or a skinny person. There are plenty of those around, so make yourself comfortable. And to those idiots who stare at you, give them a great, big warm smile. Never put an apologetic look on your face. Take the seat!

41. Try to always smell nice. People are under the illusion that big people have body odor. We all perspire and will do so at any given time. I use Dr. Bronner's magic soaps, made with organic oils. Lavender scented, pure Castile soap. Soap has numerous uses, far too many to list here. You can find this soap in any good health food store and comes in a variety of scents. This soap leaves you squeaky clean and by this, I mean you feel and hear it as you wash yourself. Don't get me wrong: I am not saying that larger people are apt to smell bad, this is only to give you a little more confidence about your cleanliness concerns. You can contact: "ALL One", Box 28, Escondido, CA 92033, *www.drbronner.com* or (760) 743-2211.

42. Give people something about which to compliment you. One of my friends has a new hairdo and she gets raves because of it. What do you think this does for her self esteem? It sends it through the roof! Isn't change the spice of life? Pick something from head to toe to change. Not everyone has a lot of money for something major. If you want a wardrobe makeover, shop in thrift stores. There are some great buys in these places. I shop on occasion in a store in Phoenix, Arizona called "My Sister's Closet" and I find great buys in my size (plus), many of which are designer fashions. Also look for novelty or specialty shops in your area for new furnishings. When you have company, you'll have nice conversation pieces around.

43. Start a collection. This will certainly get you out and about. Costume jewelry, tie clips, dolls, miniature cars, plates, teapots, whatever you like (I used to collect teapots and plates).

44. Go to garage sales, rummage sales, flea markets, if only to mix and mingle. If you want to buy something, then do so. The idea

is to keep busy, circulate and meet people. More importantly, you need the exposure. Some of the more self-conscious people need as much "other people" stimulation as possible and it's good therapy, too.

45. If you are single, then be your own date. I take me out all the time. Most of us would never entertain the idea, let alone do it. Why not? Don't you like yourself? Don't you love yourself? Be your own best company. Learn not only how to be comfortable in your own skin and body type, but also in your own company. Consider validating you. Consider pampering you. Consider being with you. Aren't you a nice person? Kind, thoughtful, endearing . . . pour on the accolades, because you deserve them. Even though we live in a so-called "two-some" or "partnered" society, there's nothing wrong with being out by oneself. I go anywhere I want alone. Besides, people will be there when I arrive, so there is always someone to talk to, even if only briefly. That's okay. I decided to move to Arizona in 2004. Someone asked me why I would move to a place where I had no family and knew no one. "Well, there will be people where I move," was my reply. How true. Now I have more friends than I can count. I am not advocating putting yourself in danger (single ladies) being by yourself. Be cautious. Be aware of your surroundings. Be out in the afternoon or in the early evening. Travel in well lighted venue. Park your car in your line of sight whenever possible. If you feel apprehensive, then ask a waiter or staff person to escort you to your vehicle. They will because it's good business. Besides, you never know when the hand of fate will smile upon you. So, dress up. Look cute. Look sensational. You married or partnered people, date more. Rekindle that torch, flame or whatever it was that brought you together in the first place. Remember what drew you together. Your waistline may have spread a little over the years and you two need reconnecting.

46. Agree to take charge and control of your choices and decisions. No one else can do this any better than you. You have your buddies to bounce things around with. Heed their advice and counsel when you find it necessary.

47. Don't consume yourself with weight loss gimmicks and fads. These things are stress producing, psychologically demoralizing and can lead to compulsive behavioral eating disorders. They place you in a revolving door cycle. You end up more frustrated and out of control. If you have any life threatening weight related issues, consult your primary care physician for alternatives.

48. Stroke yourself. Praise yourself. Tell yourself that you did good today. Tell yourself that you made the right food choices. Tell yourself that you are proud of you. Tell yourself that you have confidence in you, in your decisions and in your commitment to your overall well being. Keep yourself as upbeat as possible. This might be difficult with the everyday problems and stumbling blocks that lurk around every corner. Yet, you do possess the fortitude to hold onto you. Tell yourself that you have the innate power to change the way you look, feel, think and be. Also, rid yourself of anything antithetical to your progress. This means people who live adversely to your cause.

49. Develop a workable and doable strategy for maintenance. Use affirmations daily: I can change how I look because I have the power to do so. I ask to be more creative and devise new sources of energy. I will release negative energy from my being. I will restore the positive force within me. I am on my way to being a better self. Put affirmations like these in picture frames and read them every day when you get out of bed . . . remember that you bedroom is your sanctuary.

50. And finally, find something you believe in that enriches your soul, your spirit, your mind. No matter what age you are, expend your belief systems. Get into a religious forum, service, program. Practice and worship on a regular basis. Look to the heavens, the universe and to God for true enlightenment.

The bottom line is, folks, that you are more powerful than you think or realize. All you have to do is notice more, observe more and dream more. Your cravings and compulsions to eat and overeat are manifested in your hidden unseen selfthe self that has yet to evolve, the self that has yet to surge forward, the self that has yet to identify and let go of the past hurt, the past traumas, the past rejections, the past fears and any other past occurrences which have hindered its growth. These events are lodged deeply in the crevices of your soul, crushing your spirit and bringing about "weight pain." This is imposed upon you by something sinister, insidious and insufferable that has kept you stilted, stressed and strained beyond your control. You have been bound and chained. You need freedom only you can unleash. We need to remind ourselves that no matter what happened "ago" is gone, never to return. The memories that linger and torment us can be released by us, for us, through us, and that which we cannot release, we give over to God. We can move forward. We submit to ourselves, our true selves, to our vision of who we really want to be. We can trust in ourselves. All we need to do is let it happen and it will. The lady who says "I want a boyfriend," can have one. She needs to know that it is possible by her own efforts, not by surgery. The man who says "I want to be able to play with my grandchildren," can and should. If they really mean so much to him, then what is stopping him from losing the weight? Surgery should be used only as a last resort to save your life. But you already have that power within you. Our human selves can soar! We can become whatever we want to become. Who is stopping us? We stop ourselves. With time, we need to forgive ourselves, accept us, in our skin, in this body that we inhabit, in which we feel trapped, scared and frozen. It can melt, dissolve and redefine itself. It can quiet the storm and bring peace and calm.

Epilogue

Food—The Great Pacifier

It quiets, it lulls, it soothes, it sedates the rumbling turmoil within. Most of us were given pacifiers as babies for that reason. To keep us calm and peaceful. We were orally fixated, orally tranquilized and orally bonded and enslaved from the outset. We were staged. Out little selves would forever be embedded and entrenched in memory of what we felt as we sucked away. Those memories implanted deeply into out subconscious minds. And we'd never forget the feeling of satisfaction and euphoria. Our fingers would also provide a secondary substitute or even initial entry while in the womb.

Now the transference into adulthood has become forkfuls of sweets, delicacies. Morsels and crumbs of whatever we could get our hands on that calms that inner urge to soothe. We are like zombies, marching in trance to our pantries, closets, refrigerators, hideaways and stashes in search of pacification to assuage our pain. Oh yes, we also call it happiness, bliss, glee, cheer and the like. But it is still triggered by an emotional impetus. Unthinking and unknowing of the depth of our deep-seated destruction which has been subliminally programmed, including flashing "neon lights" proclaiming "all you can eat," "two for one," "free desserts with any two entrees," "the best all beef," "The Best Beer," "Big Mac®,' and on and on . . . . The feel better panacea that takes its form in mounds and mounds and heaps and heaps of food and calories daily, adding more and more "weight pain" to our beleaguered and embattled frames. We become contorted, misshapen, warped physically and obese more than we want to think about. We wear blinders, failing to see it coming or denying its very daily, weekly, monthly and yearly occurrence. We proceed, avoiding mirrors and go further and further into a deluge of despair, angst and pain, secretly loathing and despising what we have become or are becoming. Yet, we are powerless to stop it. Weakened, damaged, drained, daunted, disillusioned by our failings, we dangle hopelessly, quietly screaming inside ourselves. No one answers. We don't know how to help or free ourselves from this vicious circle of defeat.

But lest we forget, there is a light at the end of the road. It is our innate desire, our innate will, our innate yearning to become more of what we want to be. All we need to do is just let go; let go of the fear; let go of the "can'ts", let go of the hopelessness and allow ourselves to rise above, inch by inch, foot by foot, day by day and so on and so on. It's in there, dig down and find it. If you awaken every morning, see that as hope, see that as inspiration, see that as joy. See that as happiness and see a new vision. See it as a new opportunity to create a new you. A happier you, a healthier you. Just take one little step, no matter what it is.

Ten extra steps, lifting your arms five to ten times, smiling at your inner self in the mirror. Saying "I love you!" Saying "Oh, happy day!" Eating two strawberries with breakfast instead of whatever. Every different step you take every day will all add up eventually making a small difference, then a bigger difference you'll see but always remember to smile in the process. Never stop smiling. The time factor no longer counts and is irrelevant since each day, each added event brings new meaning and it all adds up at some point in the future. Take your time getting there. You set the pace as well as take the steps.

In the African American community, there is something we always do no matter where we are, no matter whether we know one another. That is to always say hello or smile. I guess it is a cultural thing!

So let all the "chubbets" out there from now on give a silent smile to each other, or nod, to convey that we support one another. To acknowledge that we are comrades, we are brothers and sisters, we recognize each other for who we are and we love ourselves. And we pass this on proudly.

The tabs, the "rag mags'" exploitation of women is insidious, insulting and degrading. Women gobble up every crumb, morsel and tidbit of this insanity. Every time we turn around, someone's body is plastered front and center on the cover with seemingly undesirable features: cellulite, wrinkles, flab, all the derogations of negativity that continue to send our bodies' future into oblivion, tormented by visual, frontal assaults. When is it ever going to stop?

I say ladies, let's boycott the tabs every time they degrade us, every time they parade us, every time they deny us our right to exist in our own skin. Our mothers, sisters, aunts, cousins, all femininity alike, has the right to live without assault, abuse and abrogation as deemed by the tabloids. Movie stars and our idols must be allowed to live, breathe and grow into themselves without the added pressure of "ideal size central" as perpetrated by the media. Our beautiful starlets who walk and grace the runways and red carpets should be adored for what they bring us: their talent, their charm and their allure. No matter what "package," pre-set, predetermined and not by some fashion guru who typifies what a standard of beauty is. Women must learn to accept the ideal of beauty from their own standards. They must decide on which paradigm, wants and actual desires feels good for them and to them. They must be allowed to discern and distinguish between which values appeal to them most without guilt, sadness or regret and, moreover, not to become substance abusers. Freedom of choice is a natural right which has far too long been lost in the application of pleasing oneself. To be fired or dismissed because you have gained five or ten pounds is a sacrilege, a disgrace, an injustice and a crime against humanity. How dare you?

Finally, we will always be emerging. We will always be shedding our "skin" and we will always be unveiling our newer selves, our creative selves, our dynamic selves. We must not see obesity as a curse, a weakness or a loss of faith in ourselves. We must always, always remember that each and every one of us is a champion in our own right. Why? Because we can be who and whatever we desire to be. All we need to do is ask! Ask yourself, "What do I want? What do I really want to accomplish in this life?" We need to sit down with ourselves, our true selves and weed out the damage, the pain, the heartbreak; all that which swallowed us up whole little by little, inch by inch and say, "No more, I'm done! I quit!" We can trust and allow ourselves to work it out. Never throw in the towel. As long as there is breath in our bodies there will always be hope! There will always be the light of a new day, which can bring a newer and better you.

It is my belief that people who have weight issues will come to terms with who and what they are given the freedom to do so. They need love, compassion, support and understanding, not ridicule, not torment, not leers and jeers and, above all, neither ignorance nor apathy.

For those of you who lose and regain your weight, get help. Find a weight management therapist to assist you in any weight loss program. I believe you cannot lose weight and maintain it without ongoing personal one-on-one regular, therapeutic and emotional counseling. This is an absolute must. I also believe if you can find a personal trainer, then you can find a weight management therapist. Oprah, Kirstie and all the others who yoyo, take heed.

Health care programs need to include weight loss accompanied by psychological therapy. Weight management professionals, counselors, therapists should be factored into any worthwhile weight loss programs. Health care programs must and should provide for this. Obesity is a major health concern in the U.S. and it needs to be addressed for what it actually is, a psychological eating disorder brought about by trauma, emotional stress, genetics (albeit a scientific rationale in my opinion), family lifestyle and environmental impact stemming from early childhood into adulthood.

www.ingramcontent.com/pod-product-compliance
Lightning Source LLC
Chambersburg PA
CBHW021254280526
45784CB00005B/2374